ROBERT KENNEDY'S
MUSCLEMAG *International*

AWESOME ABS!

The Gut-Busting Solution For Men & Women.

Published by MuscleMag International
6465 Airport Road
Mississauga, Ontario
Canada L4V 1E4

Designed by Jackie Kydyk

10 9 8 7 6 5 4 3 Pbk.

Canadian Cataloging in Publication Data

Chek, Paul, 1961-
    Awesome abs!: the gut-busting solution for men & women

Includes index
ISBN 1-55210-002-2

    1. Abdominal exercises. I. Title.

GV546.5.C46 1996   646.7'5   C96-900171-1

Distributed in Canada by
CANBOOK Distribution Services
1220 Nicholson Road
Newmarket, Ontario
L3Y 7V1
800-399-6858

Distributed in the United States by
BookWorld Services
1933 Whitfield Park Loop
Sarasota, Florida 34243
800-444-2524

Printed in Canada

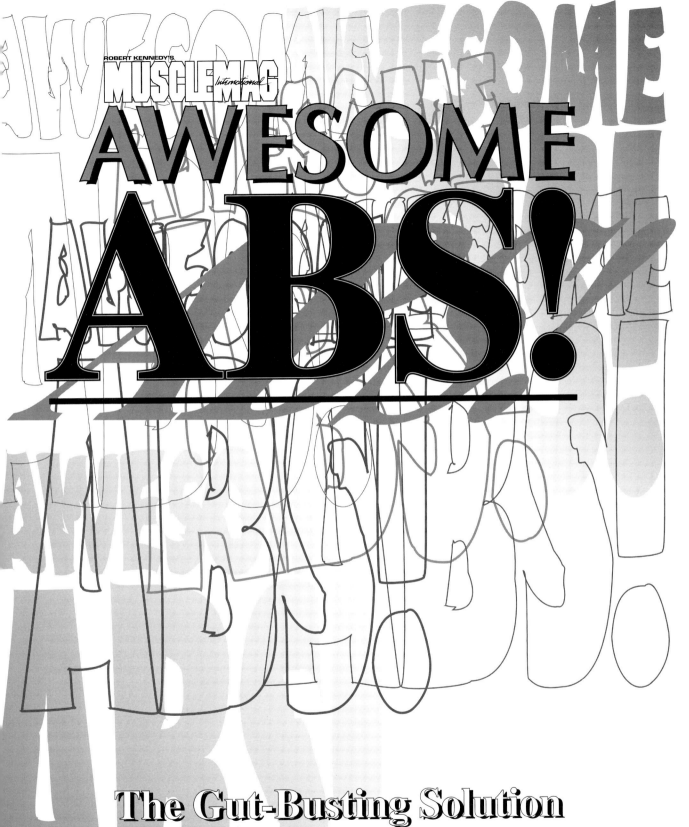

ROBERT KENNEDY'S
MUSCLEMAG *International*

AWESOME
ABS!

The Gut-Busting Solution
For Men & Women.
By Paul Chek HHP, NMT

AWESOME ABS!

– WARNING TO THE READER –

The instructions and advice contained within the pages of this book are intended for informational purposes only and are not intended as a substitute for medical counseling.

This book contains explicit information on many different exercises, training techniques and associated programs that, depending on your current physical condition and present health, may or may not prove harmful to you. Therefore, as with all exercise programs, we suggest that you consult with your doctor prior to following any of the suggestions or information contained herein.

Due care should also be given to the exercises, techniques and programs described because, if performed improperly, they may have potential to cause injury. If you feel discomfort or pain resulting from any of the exercise procedures, do not continue.

The author and publisher of this book disclaim any and all liability in connection with the exercise concepts described. The user assumes all risks while performing the exercises, techniques and programs. Use of this book implies an agreement not to bring any lawsuit or action for any injury, howsoever caused, related to its contents.

Contents

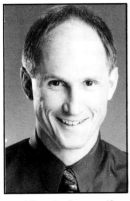

ABOUT THE AUTHOR

Paul Chek began his career as trainer of the US Army boxing team at Fort Bragg, North Carolina. While serving as a trainer of the boxing team under the guidance of team doctor Charles O. Pitluck D.O., he was able not only to implement his ideas on nutrition and training, but also to provide massage therapy for the team's fighters. After leaving the army in 1986 and moving to San Diego, California, Paul became a certified sports massage therapist. In 1989 he achieved his holistic health practitioner's certification from the Massage Training Institute in Encinitas, California. In August 1989 he completed the requirements for certification as a neuromuscular therapist through the Institute for Natural Health in St. Petersburg, Florida.

After being self-employed for two years, and working in a physical therapy clinic for four years, he became president and co-owner of Golden Triangle Rehabilitation Inc. in La Jolla, California. Currently Paul trains athletes, performs orthopedic rehabilitation, produces exercise videos and runs his seminar business from his new center, Paul Chek's Center for Health and Performance, located in La Jolla,California. Paul has contributed chapters to *Biathlon Training and Racing* by Kenny Souza and Bob Babbit, as well as *Chiropractic Approach to Head Pain,* edited by Daryl Curl. He has authored numerous articles on rehabilitation, strength training and self-help techniques for athletes. Paul holds two US patents on exercise and rehabilitation inventions, and his exercise programs and video correspondence courses are currently used by universities and professional teams in 25 countries around the world.

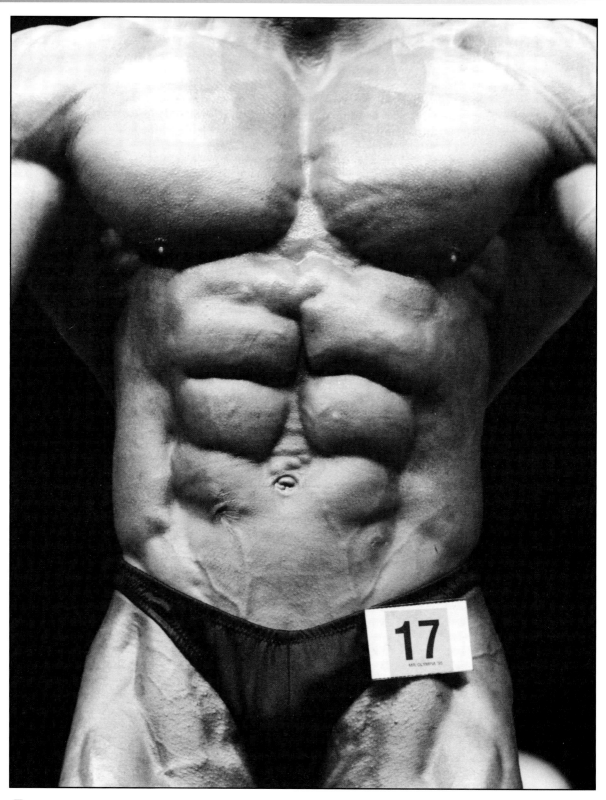

Any bodybuilder or connoisseur of the human physique will surely attest to the beauty of a washboard abdomen. Although well-defined abdominal musculature is essential to complete one's physique, size and beauty have no correlation to function.

A finely coordinated, well-conditioned abdominal region is essential for stability of the trunk, prevention of low-back pain, and maintenance of good posture. Many of the techniques used today for strengthening the upper, lower, and oblique regions of the abdomen are not functionally sound, encouraging poor posture, exacerbating old injuries, and often not exercising the intended muscles. To understand the mechanics of good technique, it is imperative that we review the functional anatomy of the abdominal region.

FUNCTIONAL ANATOMY

The abdominal musculature consists primarily of four muscles. The largest, although not the most popular, are the external obliques (Fig. 1).

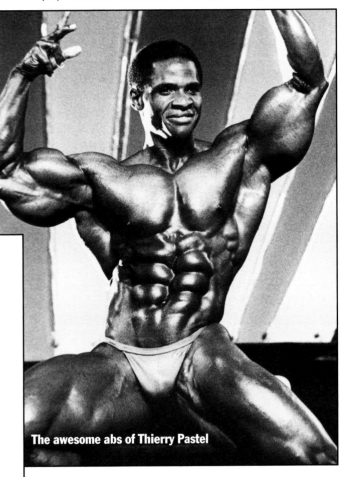

The awesome abs of Thierry Pastel

FIGURE 1

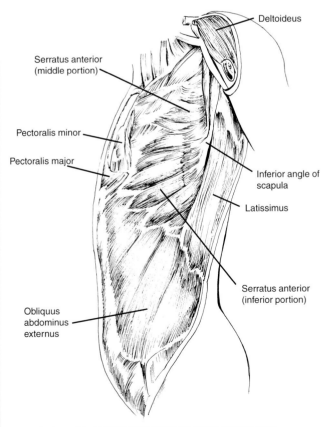

Deltoideus

Serratus anterior (middle portion)

Pectoralis minor

Pectoralis major

Inferior angle of scapula

Latissimus

Serratus anterior (inferior portion)

Obliquus abdominus externus

Anatomy pictures referenced from Sobotta *Human Anatomy*, 1906 Saunders Pub. Co. Philadelphia, PA

The internal and external obliques are trunk flexors and rotators. When the torso is to be turned left, the external oblique on the right side works synergistically with the left internal oblique, and vice versa. Between the oblique muscle groups lies the very popular rectus abdominus. The rectus abdominus serves mainly as a trunk flexor and has an important role in protecting the internal organs from external force – e.g. a boxer's punch. The transverse abdominus serves to stabilize the internal organs in a girdle-like fashion, as well as assisting in stabilization of the back via the thoracolumbar fascia. (See Fig. 2 and Fig. 7.)

FIGURE 2

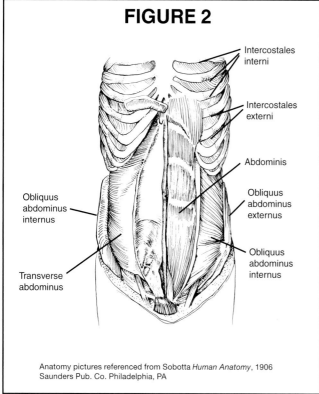

Intercostales interni

Intercostales externi

Abdominis

Obliquus abdominus internus

Obliquus abdominus externus

Obliquus abdominus internus

Transverse abdominus

Anatomy pictures referenced from Sobotta *Human Anatomy*, 1906 Saunders Pub. Co. Philadelphia, PA

FIGURE 3

Diaphragm

Medial arched ligament

Right crus

Lateral arched ligament

Left crus

Quadratus lumborum

Psoas minor

Psoas major

Iliacus

Adductor longus

Pectineus

Anatomy pictures referenced from Sobotta *Human Anatomy*, 1906 Saunders Pub. Co. Philadelphia, PA

In discussing the abdominal region, one must include the psoas and the quadratus lumborum (Fig. 3 and 4). The psoas is a primary flexor of the hip, and with the feet anchored is a powerful trunk flexor. Because most of us were brought up in school (and the military) doing situps with our feet hooked under a bench or with a partner

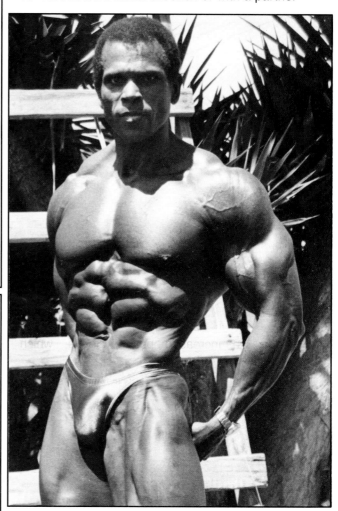

The flawless abs of France's Serge Nubret.

holding them down, we often thought that our stomach muscles were being exercised, when in reality it was chiefly our psoas muscles that were continually getting stronger. Because the psoas originates off the lumbar spine (low back) and inserts into the lesser trochanter (inner hip) , as it becomes stronger – with increased muscle tone – it brings its origin and insertion together.

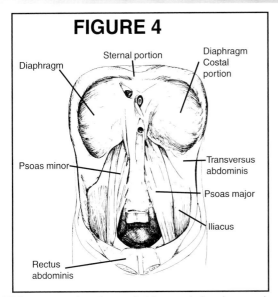

FIGURE 4

Diaphragm

Sternal portion

Diaphragm Costal portion

Psoas minor

Transversus abdominis

Psoas major

Iliacus

Rectus abdominis

This approximation of hip and lumbar spine creates increased curvature of the low back and tilts the pelvis forward, causing the pot-belly look.

Because the psoas tilts the pelvis forward, and the rectus abdominus and external obliques tilt it backward, these muscles oppose each other in this key postural function. With this in mind, I must remind you of Davis's Law, which states: If muscle ends are brought closer together, there occurs an increased pull of tonus, which shortens the muscle and may even cause hypertrophy (increased size). If muscle ends are separated beyond normal, tonus is lessened or lost with the result that the muscle may become weak. Any exercise that is intended to strengthen the abdominal muscles, but which, because of poor technique, strengthens the psoas muscles instead, will not only tip the pelvis forward, displacing the centre of gravity forward and altering posture, but will also encourage weakening of the abdominal muscles (especially relative to psoas strength).

With the pelvis tipped forward the body must compensate by leaning the trunk backward and the head forward in an attempt to stay vertical. This movement causes increased pressure in the small joints of the lumbar spine (facet joints), which can cause an inflammatory response and back pain. The forward head is commonly associated with neck pain and headaches. (See

Fig. 5 showing pelvic tilt and forward head.)

The quadratus lumborum (Fig. 3) is the deepest muscle of the low back and is also considered part of the abdominal wall. This muscle is heavily used in side lying situps and is commonly the cause of low-back pain after such

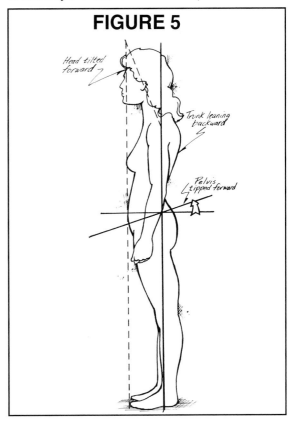

FIGURE 5

Head tilted forward

Trunk leaning backward

Pelvis tipped forward

As the pelvis tips forward, the head often comes forward proportionally. This reaction may be seen as a result of a strength imbalance between the psoas and abdominal musculature. The long-term implications of such postural changes are reduced athletic performance, higher susceptibility to injury, and perpetual imbalance of length-tension relationships between muscle groups. For the bodybuilder this means poor symmetry.

exercises. Because of this risk I recommend that those with a history of back injury avoid this exercise and start with standing dumbell side flexions. Begin with standing torso side bends, holding a dumbell in the opposite hand. Use a weight you can perform 15-20 reps with and increase the resistance to an 8-12 rep load over 8-12 weeks before attempting a side lying situp.

11

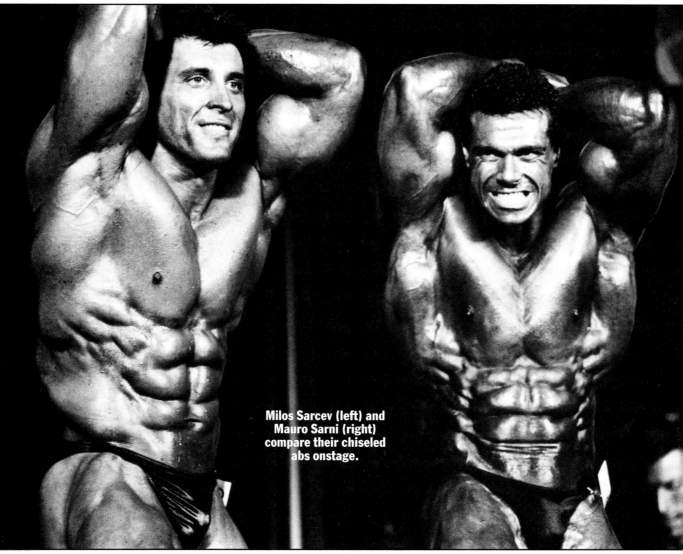

Milos Sarcev (left) and
Mauro Sarni (right)
compare their chiseled
abs onstage.

ABDOMINAL SUPPORT MECHANISMS OF THE LOWER BACK

An essential function of the abdominal muscu- lature is to provide support for the low back. The two primary means of accomplishing this task are 1) through intra-abdominal pressure (hy- draulic support), and 2) thoracolumbar fascia gain.

Intra-abdominal pressure is created by contraction of the abdominal muscles against the viscera (internal organs). Because the viscera are encapsulated by the diaphragm above and the pelvic basin below, any contraction of the abdominal wall forces the viscera both upward and downward into these barriers. As the viscera are displaced upward into the diaphragm (especially when the breath is held or on resisted exhalation), there is a traction force placed on the lumbar spine. This traction force, referred to as the hydraulic support mechanism, is believed to alleviate as much as 30 percent of the load on the lumbar spine. The commonly heard hissing, growling, grunting and yelling coming from those performing heavy lifts is a way of contracting the

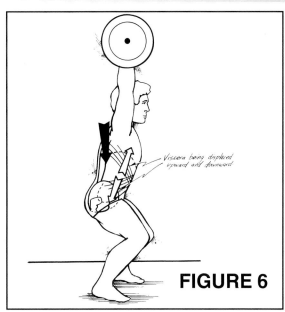

Viscera being displaced upward and downward

FIGURE 6

As the abdominal musculature contracts during a lifting effort, the internal organs are pushed into the diaphragm above and the pelvic basin below (as shown by the two white arrows). This shift creates a lifting mechanism, reducing the pressure through the lower lumbar vertebrae (low back). The black arrow indicates the pressure through the low back during a lift.

abdominal wall and tensing the diaphragm against the rising viscera, creating an effective lift mechanism to protect the lumbar discs from rupture. As the weight one attempts to lift increases, so too will one's need for abdominal strength (Fig. 6). Interestingly, weight belts have been shown to increase intra-abdominal pressure. *Unfortunately, when a weight belt is used, the brain will not activate the abdominal muscles to their full potential.* For this reason weight belts should be worn only for maximum lifts. Weight belts can alter the normal mechanics of your lumbar spine (especially when worn tightly). Their use may lead to breakdown in the lower lumbar discs.

The dense layer of connective tissue in the low back is known as thoracolumbar fascia. Through its attachments to the spine the transverse abdominus and a few fibers of the internal oblique provide crucial support for the low back. Because the posterior layer of thoracolumbar fascia has two laminae that form a diamond-shaped vector, lateral traction by the transverse abdominus and internal oblique create a force that resists flexion (forward bending) of the lumbar spine, thus giving it support during lifting movements that would tend to force flexion of the low back. The force of this resistance to flexion of the lumbar spine is said to be about 57 percent of the lateral force created by the abdominal muscles, and is called the thoracolumbar fascia gain. (See Fig. 7.)

FIGURE 7

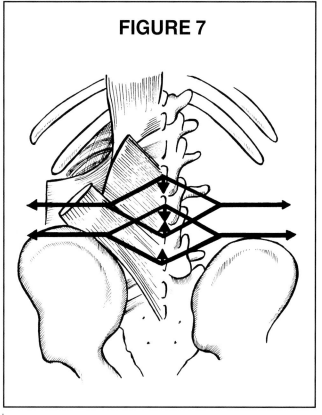

The fiber armament of the thoracolumbar fascia is such that a contraction of the internal oblique and transverse abdominus muscles will create an extension or backward-bending force. The lateral force generated by these muscles is indicated by the arrows pointing away from the spine; the backward-bending force created by this pull is shown by the arrows along the spine. This backward-bending force is referred to by Bogduk as thoracolumbar fascia gain.

Modified from *Clinical Anatomy of the Lumbar Spine* by Bogduk & Twomey Publisher: Churchill Livingstone, 1987 ISBN 0-443-03505-9

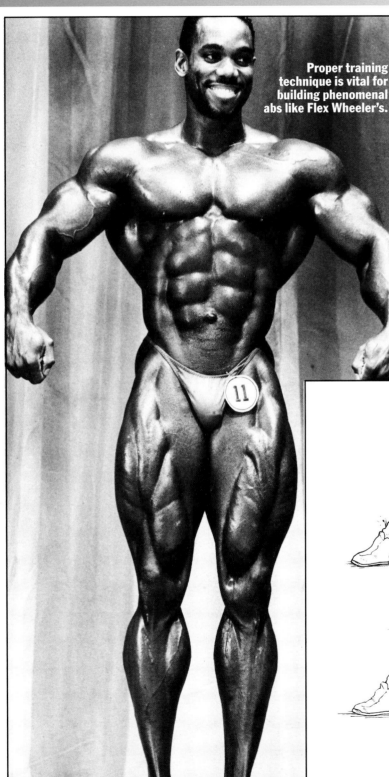

Proper training technique is vital for building phenomenal abs like Flex Wheeler's.

TRAINING TECHNIQUE
• KNOW WHERE TO BEGIN

Prior to beginning any abdominal conditioning program, coordination should be assessed. One commonly finds bodybuilders and athletes of the most elite levels with very strong upper abdominals, weak lower abdominals, and poor coordination. Poor coordination represents undirected strength, once again predisposing the back to injury.

When I speak of abdominal coordination, I am referring to the lower abdominal

Lying flat on your back as shown, preferably on a firm surface, roll your pelvis backward, flattening your back against the floor. Hold pressure against the floor for 10 seconds; relax and repeat. This exercise should be done for two minutes or to fatigue, up to six times per day.

FIGURE 8
Supine Pelvic Tilt – Exercise 1

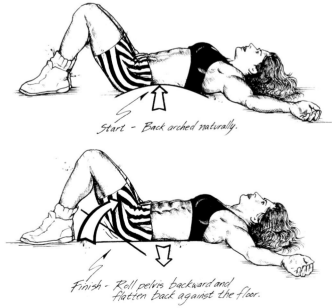

Start - Back arched naturally.

Finish - Roll pelvis backward and flatten back against the floor.

FIGURE 9
Supine Pelvic Tilt – Single Leg – Exercise 2

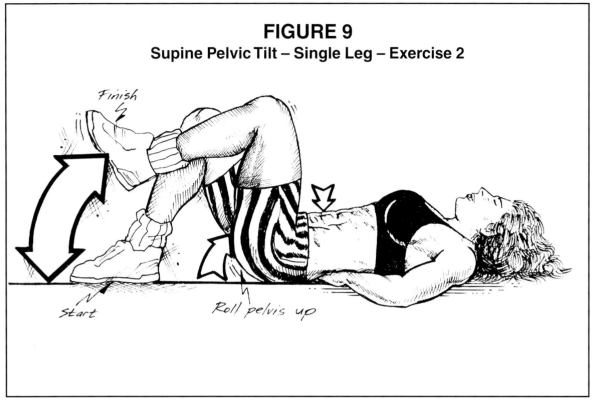

With knees bent and feet flat on the floor, roll your pelvis backward until your spine presses firmly against your fingers as shown. While holding pressure against your fingers, raise and lower your leg as demonstrated. Alternate left and right until your ability to keep your back against your fingers diminishes. For maximum results perform multiple sets of less than two minutes in duration.

musculature's ability to stabilize the pelvis and lumbar curvature while simultaneously contracting or relaxing the psoas muscle. This is particularly important because if the abdominal muscles do not effectively maintain good posture of the pelvis, allowing the psoas to tilt it forward, there will be a progressive increase in the curvature of the spine, leading to postural degeneration. (See Fig. 5 showing symmetry between pelvic tilt and forward head.) This postural degeneration will lead to a perpetuation of imbalance in the length/tension relationships of many opposing muscle groups, disturbing the symmetry that all bodybuilders work for.

The ability to hold one's back flat against the floor while steadily lowering the legs is required as normal coordination. If one cannot achieve this capability, exercises 1 and 2 are your beginning point for both coordination and lower-abdominal strengthening (Fig. 8 and 9). Once you have mastered these two, you are ready to attempt the coordination test (exercise number 3, Fig. 10). After passing the coordination test with the legs fully relaxed at the knees, you can begin to open the angle at the knee (Fig. 11). This variation proportionally increases the weight of the legs, the pull of the psoas, and thus the load on the lower abdomen in its efforts to keep the back stabilized. At this point exercise number 4 (Fig. 12) may be used for strengthening the lower abdomen.

Many people experience back pain while doing abdominal exercises. If after reading this book you find that your technique has been correct, but you still have back pain with exercises, you must stretch the low-back and psoas musculature prior to beginning exercises. If you find that your technique has been

15

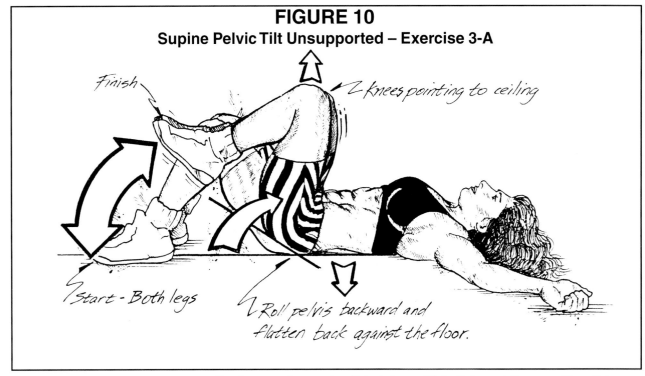

FIGURE 10
Supine Pelvic Tilt Unsupported – Exercise 3-A

Finish

knees pointing to ceiling

Start - Both legs

Roll pelvis backward and flatten back against the floor.

This exercise is the same as coordination exercise number 2, but done with both legs at the same time. It is also a coordination test. Normal coordination between the psoas and abdominal musculature is such that you should be able to hold your back against the floor (or your fingers) while simultaneously lowering your feet to the floor.

incorrect, you must first make the necessary changes in technique, as well as stretching before your ab workout. Stretching the commonly shortened hyperactive lumbar and psoas muscles helps relax them, letting the intended muscle do the work. The book titled *Stretching* by Bob Anderson is a good place to start if you have no stretching routine.

If you sit all day at work, you may actually have

Once you have mastered exercise 3-A, you can begin to open the angle at the knee. This lengthening of the leg increases the load placed upon the psoas to hold the leg up. Proportionally more strength from the lower abs is required to keep the back flat against the floor. You must never let your back rise off the floor or your hands, as this movement only reinforces the pattern you're trying to break! The ability to keep the back flat and lower the legs (bent and relaxed at the knee) is considered a sign of good coordination.

a flat back. This condition can be determined by standing with your heels, seat, back and head against a wall. If you cannot slide the fingers and palm of your hand between the wall and your back, you are probably in need of more curve in your low back. If this is the case, you are more

FIGURE 11 – Exercise 3-B

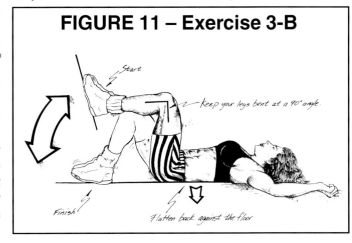

Start

keep your legs bent at a 90° angle.

Finish

Flatten back against the floor

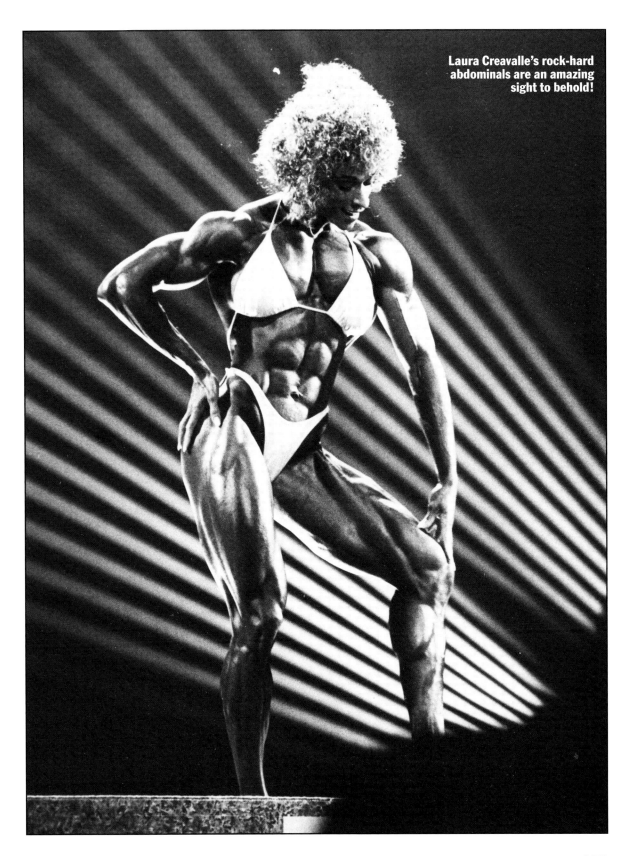

Laura Creavalle's rock-hard abdominals are an amazing sight to behold!

likely to benefit from hip flexion exercises and should consult a physical therapist. The cable crunch can be performed by adding hip flexion at the completion of the crunch phase for the flat-bench exerciser. This technique will encourage psoas use and helps restore the natural curve to your back. If indeed you have a flat back and seem to continue to get back pain with abdominal exercises, I recommend consultation with a physical therapist. Remember that regardless of the curve in your low back (excessive or reduced), the coordination exercises must be mastered to ensure normal dynamic stabilization in the low back and pelvis.

I recall working with a patient who was suffering form a substantial low-back injury (spondylolisthesis) from deadlifting. Upon testing his abdominal coordination and finding it to be very poor, he was surprised how well exercise number 4 isolated the low abs. Although exercise 4 (Fig. 12) seemed very simple on paper, he was amazed to find that he could do only a few repetitions before being fatigued. After a total revision of his abdominal program, and some postural training, he now claims a 90 percent reduction in pain.

TRAINING ORDER

After determining your level of coordination, and starting at your level of ability, strengthening of the lower, oblique, and upper abdominal regions should begin. First the lower abs should be exercised, followed by the obliques, and then the upper abs. This order is recommended because the lower abs and obliques require the most coordinated movement patterns, both needing support from the generally stronger upper abdominals. After successfully training the lower ab and oblique regions, you can exercise the upper abs. With that sequence in mind let's begin with the lower abdominals.

Lying on your back, knees pointed upward and hips flexed to 90°, pretend that your knees have strings attaching them to the ceiling. As you roll your pelvis back – flattening your back – imagine that the strings are being pulled as though you were a puppet. Try to get your knees to rise a half-inch, allowing only vertical movement of the thighs. Placing the arms above the head helps counterbalance the weight of the lower body. Try to keep the neck relaxed and breathe with the belly. It's not as easy as it looks!

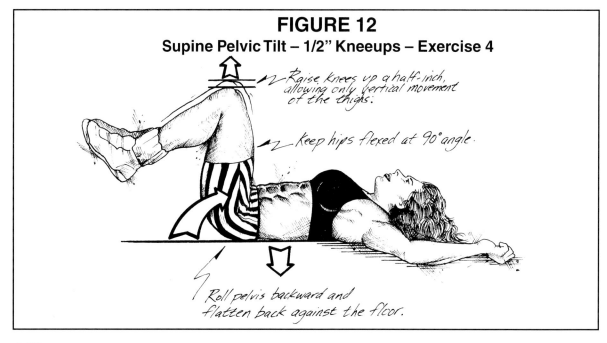

FIGURE 12
Supine Pelvic Tilt – 1/2" Kneeups – Exercise 4

Raise knees up a half-inch, allowing only vertical movement of the thighs.

Keep hips flexed at 90° angle.

Roll pelvis backward and flatten back against the floor.

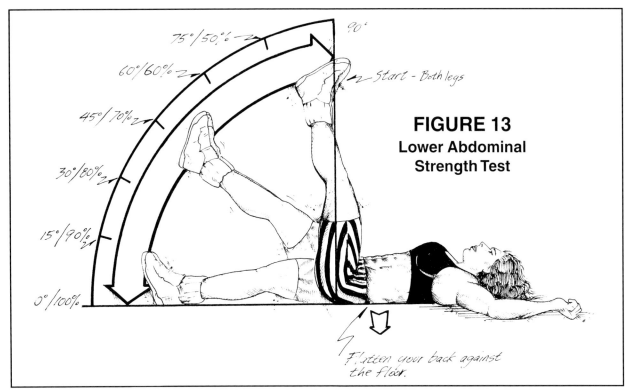

75°/50%
90°
60/60%
Start – Both legs
45°/70%

FIGURE 13
Lower Abdominal
Strength Test

30°/80%

15°/90%

0°/100%

Flatten your back against the floor.

The lower abdominal strength test is virtually the same as exercise 3, with the legs now straightened. Place either your fingers (or a partner's) under your low back at belly-button level. Begin with the legs at 90° or straight up in the air as shown. At this point roll the pelvis back, placing pressure on your fingers. From here lower your legs without allowing the low back to rise off the floor (or substantially decreasing the pressure on the fingers). The point at which your back begins to rise will be indicative of your present lower abdominal strength, as indicated on the chart. For adult males 100 percent is the ability to lower your legs to the floor without letting the back rise. Adult females should be able to lower their legs to 30° before their back begins to rise. (Good luck!)
Modified from *Muscles: Testing and Function* Third ed.
By F.P. Kendall and E. Kendall-McCreary
Publisher: Williams and Wilkins, 1983

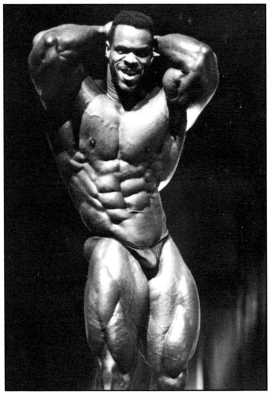

Big Paul Dillett squeezes his incredible abs onstage.

LOWER ABDOMINAL TRAINING EXERCISES

The lower abdomen, although very important to normal posture, appears to be the least understood by bodybuilders and fitness enthusiasts alike. Most individuals begin their lower-ab program using exercises that a) primarily stress the psoas, b) are far too demanding, and c) require complex movement patterns that they cannot perform.

The reverse crunch places the initial load on the lower abdominal musculature as the pelvis is rotated backward. After about 10° of posterior rotation the work load is progressively transferred upward through the abdominal muscles. The start position in fig. 14 requires that the hips be flexed until the back *begins* to flatten on the floor. (Do not flex hips until curve in low back is gone – only to the point it *begins* to flatten.) This technique has an inhibitory effect on the psoas. The arms are commonly placed above the head for counterbalancing weight. From the start position in fig. 15 the pelvis is rolled backward like a wheel until the abdominal musculature is fully contracted, and no farther! The knees cannot be used as a reference point as to how far to go because people have different torso lengths. If the legs are taken past the point of full abdominal contraction, strain will inevitably be placed on the neck!

Australia's Lee Priest flexes
his supertight abdominals.

FIGURE 14
Reverse Crunch

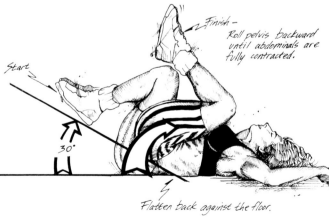

Start

Finish –
Roll pelvis backward
until abdominals are
fully contracted.

30°

Flatten back against the floor.

A prerequisite to choosing a strengthening exercise is to master the coordination exercises. Coordination exercise number 3 becomes a strengthening exercise as you increase the angle of the knee from fully relaxed toward straight leg. After you have reached 100 percent lower abdominal strength, and can stabilize your pelvis and low back, you are ready to progress to more demanding routines. Normal or 100 percent lower abdominal strength for adult males is achieved when you are able to hold your back flat on the floor while lowering your legs from 90° to 0°; adolescents and adult females should be able to lower their legs to 30° (80 percent). As shown in Fig. 13, the point at which your back rises off the floor is indicative of your current level of strength. Exercise number 4 can be utilized for strengthening as soon as you are able to perform the movement with no flexion or extension of the hips – only vertical movement.

After you have reached a level of proficiency in coordination exercises 1-4, the reverse crunch can be implemented. (See Fig. 14 and 15.) This exercise can be performed on an incline for increased resistance. The granddaddy of the lower abdominal exercises is the vertical or hanging reverse crunch. (See Fig. 16.) Unfortunately I see people attempting this

FIGURE 15
Reverse Crunch on Incline

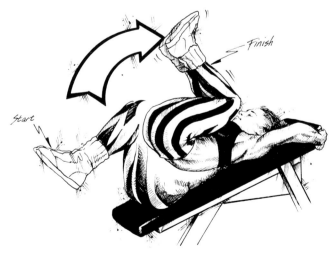

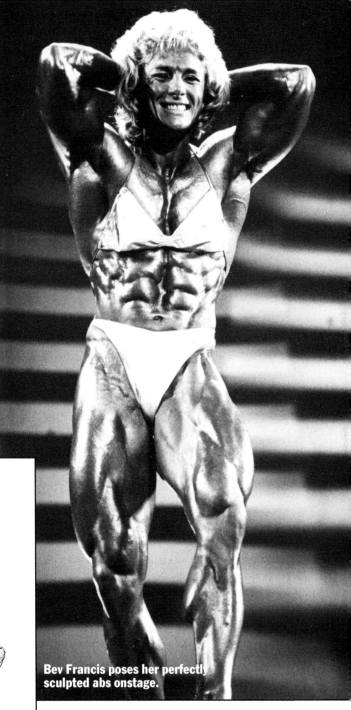

Bev Francis poses her perfectly sculpted abs onstage.

exercise with very poor form and far less than normal lower abdominal strength, leading to strong recruitment of the psoas and continued postural degeneration.

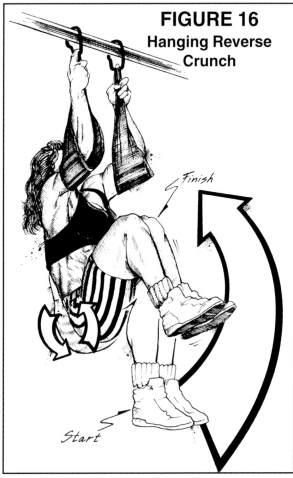

FIGURE 16
Hanging Reverse Crunch

After one has mastered the reverse crunch on a horizontal surface, and then on the incline, and has 100 percent lower abdominal strength – and only then – should the hanging reverse crunch be attempted. The legs are flexed at the hip until the curve just begins to come out of the low back (as determined by a spotter). This discourages contraction of the psoas through a poor length / tension relationship. With the hips locked in this position, the pelvis is rotated backward like a wheel (a movement which can only be done by the lower abdominal musculature) until the abdominal muscles are fully contracted.When the exercise is performed with proper technique as illustrated here, inertia from throwing the legs is eliminated, the abdominal musculature is isolated, and the stud factor is high!

WARNING: Done with poor technique, this exercise is often harmful to the low back.

THE OBLIQUES: TRAINING AND TECHNIQUE

The obliques are very important muscles, serving as our primary trunk rotators. Equally important is the postural function of the anterior (front) fibers of the external obliques, as they allow us to keep our pelvis positioned in neutral while the rectus abdominus relaxes during inspiration (breathing in). If the rectus abdominus is held tight (as it often is for the hard

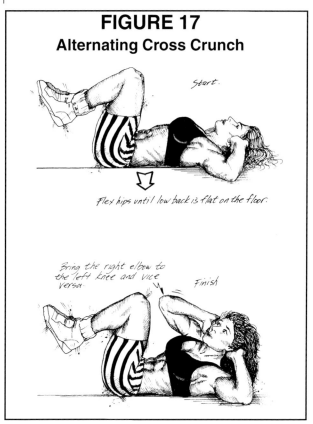

FIGURE 17
Alternating Cross Crunch

Before beginning this exercise, it is imperative that you review the section titled Crunch Technique. With the hips flexed until the low back begins to flatten, the crunch is initiated, bringing the right elbow toward the left knee and vice versa. The crunch is complete when the oblique muscles are fully contracted, not necessarily when the elbow touches the knee as often believed. The exercise can be executed right to left and left to right to the point of fatigue, or you can go to the point of fatigue on one side and then the other.

look), as the diaphragm drops with inspiration, the viscera (internal organs) have nowhere to go. This restriction inhibits normal respiratory movement of the diaphragm and rib cage, encouraging chest breathing, which requires additional work of the accessory muscles of respiration. Because hypertrophy (thickening) of accessory respiratory muscles encourages a forward head posture, this too can cause posture to degenerate from the top down, leading to a posture like that shown in Fig. 5.

FIGURE 18
Cross Crunch with Pelvic Rotation

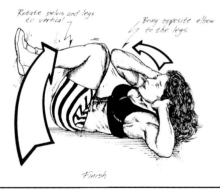

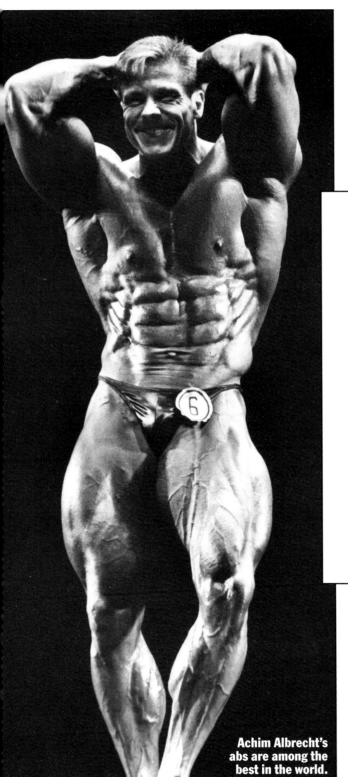

Achim Albrecht's abs are among the best in the world.

This advanced oblique exercise requires extensive rotation in the low back and should be cleared by your doctor if you have back problems past or present. Beginning with the hips flexed to the same point at which your low back begins to flatten, allow the pelvis and legs to rotate until the legs rest on the floor, never permitting the hip angle to change. Begin the exercise by rotating the pelvis and legs toward neutral (vertical) while simultaneously performing a cross crunch, or bringing the opposite elbow to the legs. This exercise is best done to fatigue on one side and then the other.

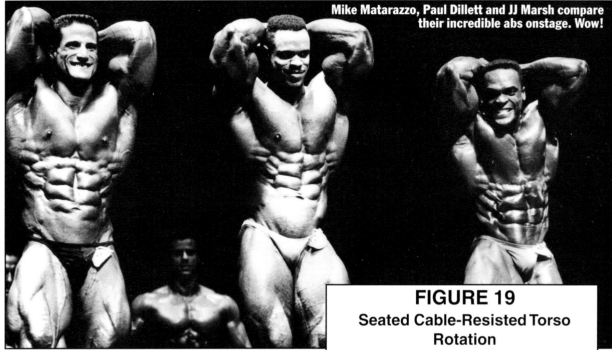

Mike Matarazzo, Paul Dillett and JJ Marsh compare their incredible abs onstage. Wow!

The cable-resisted torso rotation is an exercise commonly used to provide higher resistance than can be achieved through floor exercises. With the bench facing away from the weight stack at 45°, seat yourself and support the cable handle on your chest. From the start position, rotate and slightly flex the trunk until your shoulders are square with the bench.

The alternating cross crunch (Fig. 17) is a modified crunch which emphasizes torso rotation. Prior to beginning any crunch exercise, you should review proper technique for positioning the head and back as described in the section titled Crunch Technique.

The cross crunch with pelvic counterrotation (Fig. 18) is an outstanding exercise which works the obliques through their full range of motion. This exercise is not advised for those with a back condition, unless approved by your doctor. Any exercise that induces rotation to the lumbar spine may initiate, perpetuate, and/or exacerbate damage in lumbar discs. This warning applies to rotary torso machines as well.

The seated cable-resisted torso rotations and supine (lying on your back) cable-resisted lower-body rotation are modifications of the above

FIGURE 19
Seated Cable-Resisted Torso Rotation

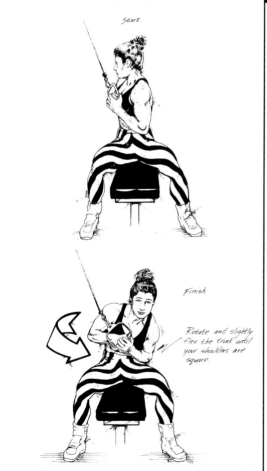

Start

Finish

Rotate and slightly flex the trunk until your shoulders are square.

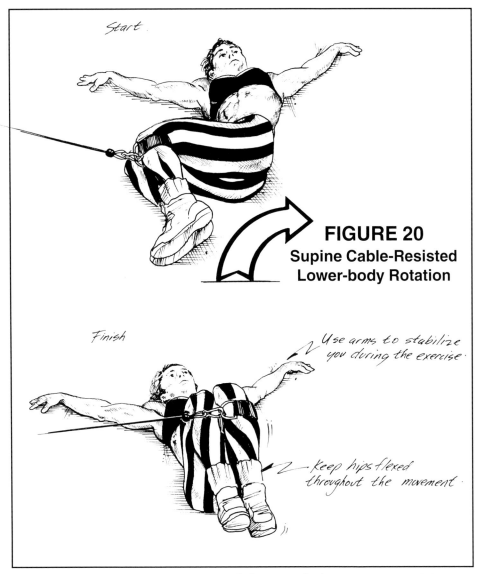

Start

FIGURE 20
Supine Cable-Resisted Lower-body Rotation

Finish

Use arms to stabilize you during the exercise.

Keep hips flexed throughout the movement.

The start position is the same as for the cross crunch with pelvic counterrotation shown in Fig. 18. The resistance is provided by the bottom pulley and cable (standard to most pulley machines). Stabilization is needed from the arms while the legs and pelvis rotate away from the machine, finishing the motion. For stability of the low back keep the hips flexed as you drop them to the start position again.

these positions. If for instance you can sit up with your arms reaching out but not across your chest, then you should begin at level 1 – i.e. arms reaching out. The next level of resistance beyond hands to head is the incline bench, followed

exercises that allow the use of increased resistance for bodybuilders (Figs. 19 and 20).

by adding weight to the chest, and finally by being weighted on an incline.

Holding 25- or 35-pound plates behind your head during crunch exercises is not advisable. As the abdominal muscles fatigue, inevitably you begin to pull on the plate in the struggle, hyperflexing your neck. This hyperflexion of the neck encourages sprain of the lower cervical spine and strain of the neck extensors, thereby promoting cervical dysfunction. The resulting discomfort can be avoided by placing a dumbell on your chest and utilizing good form, as outlined below under Crunch Technique.

THE UPPER ABDOMEN
• DETERMINING THE APPROPRIATE LEVEL OF RESISTANCE

There are three standard levels of resistance for those beginning an abdominal program. They are 1) arms reaching out, 2) arms crossed on chest, and 3) hands to head. To determine where to start your program, simply lie on your back and attempt to sit up with arms in each of

AWESOME ABS!

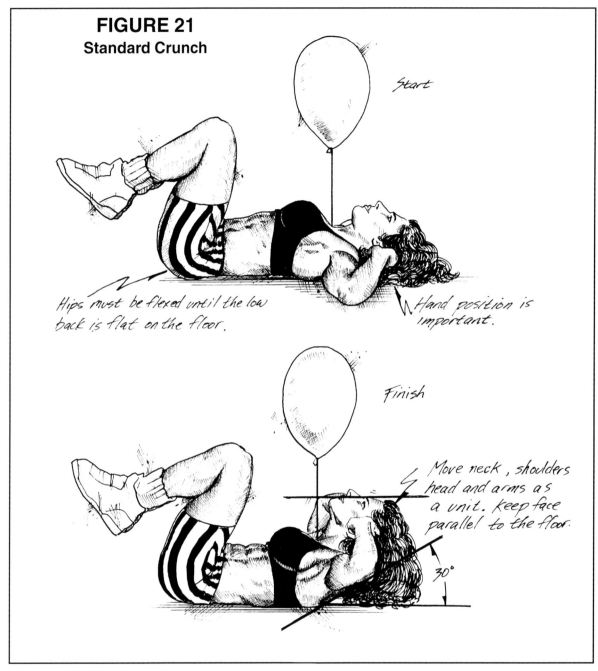

FIGURE 21
Standard Crunch

Start

Hips must be flexed until the low back is flat on the floor.

Hand position is important.

Finish

Move neck, shoulders head and arms as a unit. Keep face parallel to the floor.

30°

To begin, the hips must be flexed until the low back begins to flatten, reducing any contribution from the psoas and stabilizing the low back. Hand placement and the tongue position are crucial to proper form, as discussed in the section titled Crunch Technique. The crunch is initiated without any pulling on the head, while moving the neck, shoulders, head and arms as a unit. Imagining that you're being lifted by a helium balloon from the sternum (chest bone) helps to visualize proper motion. The crunch motion is complete when the abdominal muscles are fully contracted – no sooner, no later. To protect the neck from excess strain, the cervical curvature is maintained by keeping the face parallel to the ceiling as shown here.

26

CRUNCH TECHNIQUE

The crunch (Fig. 21), by far the most common abdominal exercise today, can be seen being performed incorrectly in almost any gym, often by people with so-called instructor certification. In the hands-to-head position the fingers should never be interlocked, but should rest gently behind the ears, without pulling. The head's center of gravity is said to be in the middle of the head at the level of the auditory meatus (ear hole). Holding behind the head with interlocked fingers encourages pulling on the head as you fatigue, and hand position is commonly above the level of the ears, increasing the leverage of the head on the neck, encouraging strain.

Because the cervical flexors tend to be weak postural muscles, and the forward head is a universally common postural fault, the neck flexors should be allowed to help support the head. *The key component to properly utilizing the cervical flexors is proper placement of the tongue in its physiological rest position, which is against the roof of the mouth just behind the* front teeth. Next, care must be taken not to lead the crunch with the head (like an ostrich), as this practice promotes a forward head posture. To break the habit of leading the crunch with your head, imagine that you have a large helium balloon attached to your sternum (chest bone) just below the collar bones. With this picture in mind try to initiate the crunch from the sternum

Like the hanging reverse crunch, this exercise is frequently done with poor technique, giving the false impression that the upper abs are being exercised. In reality the psoas is doing most of the work if you bend from the hip. The cable should come from behind as shown below and the arms should be held firmly to the trunk for stability. The seat should be tucked under to help stabilize the low back. The crunch is then performed from the top down, one vertebra at a time, until the rectus abdominus is fully contracted, and no more. Any further forward bending past this point must come from hip flexion, requiring psoas contraction, again getting away from abdominal isolation.

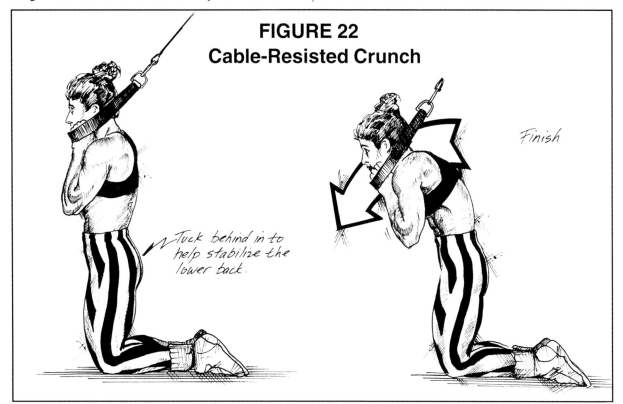

FIGURE 22
Cable-Resisted Crunch

Tuck behind in to help stabilize the lower back.

Finish

as though you were being pulled by the balloon.

The eyes should be fixed on a spot on the ceiling, the face kept parallel to the ceiling, and the head maintained as close as possible to neutral alignment (ear in line with shoulder) while the crunch is executed. This alignment encourages maintenance of the neck's natural curvature. There should be only enough lift on the head from the hands to balance the head, allowing the cervical flexors to get some needed exercise. If your neck gets sore and your tongue has been in position, there is nothing to worry about. Your neck flexors just need to catch up with your stomach muscles.

To protect your low back, the hips should be flexed until your low back just begins to flatten. In this way you keep the joints of the lumbar spine in a loose-packed or rest position and inhibit the psoas, allowing the abdominal muscles to do the work. As you execute the crunch, there should be no movement of the thighs – i.e. recruitment of the psoas. *Whenever possible avoid using bulky or overly soft mats for abdominal work.* Using only enough padding to protect the bony prominences of the back allows increased sense of body position, preventing degeneration of proper form.

Normal range of motion for the rectus abdominus in trunk flexion is approximately 30°. This means that the rectus abdominus is fully contracted shortly after the shoulder blades leave the floor. The torso should be allowed to come all the way back until the shoulder blades touch the floor again, as this represents one full repetition. Baby crunches exercise the muscle in less than physiological range of motion and are improper technique. An example of the baby crunch would be only half of a biceps curl. Executing crunches past the point at which the rectus abdominus is fully contracted, and premature use of increased resistance, encourage not only pulling on your neck for leverage but also throwing your thighs to counterbalance your torso.

The pace at which you repeat your crunches is variable depending on your purpose. If you are trying to build bulk with high resistance (added weight or incline), a slow tempo of three seconds concentric, three seconds eccentric with a weight allowing 8-12 reps is optimal. For endurance-building sets, where you may be doing 20 to 100 reps, full range of motion and good rhythm are essential.

The cable machines can be utilized to do crunch exercises, but require close attention to form in order to avoid psoas involvement (Fig. 22). The only time the psoas should be exercised is

FIGURE 23
Stretching

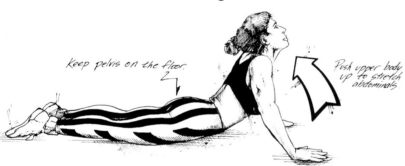

Keep pelvis on the floor.

Push upper body up to stretch abdominals

Lying prone as though you were about to do a pushup, keep the pelvis on the floor and push up. Once you feel a good stretch in the abdominal muscles, take a deep belly breath, stretching them even further. To get the stretch into the oblique muscles, rotate the torso to one side. The stretch will be through the obliques on the side which you're looking away from. Hold the stretch for at least 20 seconds in each position while breathing deeply. This abdominal stretch is a must after all ab workouts.

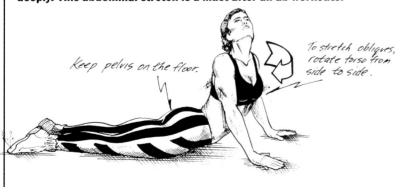

Keep pelvis on the floor.

To stretch obliques, rotate torso from side to side.

when you have developed adequate abdominal strength to maintain normal postural position of the pelvis, and/or have reduced lumbar curve (as determined by your doctor or a physical therapist). The psoas gets plenty of exercise from walking, running, jumping and activities of daily life unless you are a sedentary person, in which case postural balance of psoas vs. abdomen is to be determined by a trained therapist.

CRUNCH MACHINES

Because of the great diversity of body size among individuals and between sexes, the abdominal machines generally fit only the people in the middle ranges. There is nothing that can be accomplished on an abdominal machine that can't be accomplished through the preceding exercises. Few people know how – or even take the time – to set the machines up properly with the result that poor form leading to strain and often to back pain is common. If you should choose to use an abdominal machine, you would be well advised to have a professional fitness trainer teach you proper set-up. Because many crunch machines have foot straps, and because too high a weight is often selected, the psoas and even the quadratus lumborum may be recruited, encouraging back pain.

MYTHS OF ABDOMINAL TRAINING

There are three common myths of abdominal training. The first is that doing abdominal exercises will remove fat from your abdomen. This is not true unless, of course, you can do crunches for 30 minutes a day in your target heart-rate zone! The body, as nicely described by Covert Bailey in the book *Fit or Fat*, has its own genetic code for removing fat stores from various locations. Thus some men have big, fat beer bellies but lean, strong-looking legs, and some women can never seem to get rid of their lumpy behinds or chunky thighs.

The second myth is that you should train your abdominal muscles every day. This too is false. For a period of time you can get away with daily submaximal performances until you decondition

to that level. The only way daily ab-training should be performed is on a split routine – for example, Monday lower abs, Tuesday obliques, Wednesday upper abs. The abdominal muscles are striated skeletal muscle, just like any other muscle you exercise in the gym. You wouldn't do heavy leg extensions, triceps, biceps, or deltoid work every day of the week, would you? Micro trauma from hard exercise takes from 24 to 72 hours to repair, so if you're in a building phase,

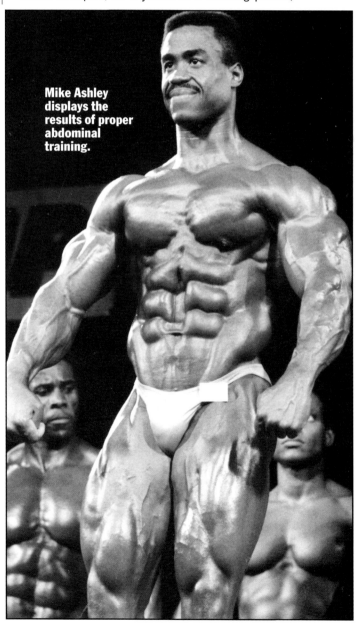

Mike Ashley displays the results of proper abdominal training.

time off between sessions is necessary. Remember this rule: Work them hard and rest them hard!

The third myth is that flutter kicks and leg extensions strengthen the lower abdomen. The truth is that they stress the lower abdominal muscles only indirectly. During flutter kicks and leg extensions the lower abs' primary job is to maintain the postural position of the pelvis against the pull of the psoas and hip flexors of the thigh (rectus femoris sartorius tensor fascia lata) which are holding most of the weight of the legs. This is why there are a lot more stresses on the lower abs with the legs straight (longer lever arm) than bent. It is apparent then that, if the low back rises off the floor, the lower abs are either being overloaded or they're not working. The burn you think is coming from your abs is really your psoas. Sorry!

SHORT- AND LONG-TERM IMPLICATIONS OF POOR TECHNIQUE

The fact should be growing ever so clear at this point that, because of the postural significance of this very important muscle group, training the abdominal muscles with poor technique has far-reaching implications. The short-term implications are generally 1) poor results, 2) a higher likelihood of causing or exacerbating a cervical or back injury, 3)

headaches, and 4) initiating a process of postural degeneration.

The long-term implications are 1) poor results, 2) development of a postural injury to the back, neck, shoulder, or even in an extremity if left long enough, 3) headaches, 4) perpetuation of poor neuromuscular motor programs and altered biomechanics, 5) decreased sports performance and increased chance of injury, and 6) increased aches and pains with slowed recovery from exercise.

PUTTING IT ALL TOGETHER
•BEGINNER'S PROGRAM

An effective abdominal program begins with coordination development, followed by strengthening exercises for the lower, then oblique, and finally upper abdominal regions. The strength-building exercises should be done to the point of fatigue no more than every other day, while coordination exercises can be done daily.

All who choose to administer an effective abdominal program, regardless of their personal level of fitness, should master the coordination exercises. When 20 repetitions of each coordination exercise can be performed (beginning with number 1), you can effectively progress to the next one. Once you have mastered 1 through 3, number 3 can be done periodically (once or twice per week) as a tune-up to maintain the nervous system's memory of this good program. Coordination exercise 4 is a useful strengthening exercise, but you must develop the coordination to use it as such.

The beginner is advised to start with only one set to fatigue of each strengthening exercise – i.e. one exercise for each region of the abdomen. When you're able to complete an abdominal workout with only minimal or no soreness the following day, you are ready to add a second set. The same principle can be used for the addition of a third set. The intermediate and advanced-level participant may work the strength exercises to failure.

FIGURE 24
Weighted Crunch on Horizontal Plane – Legs Unsupported

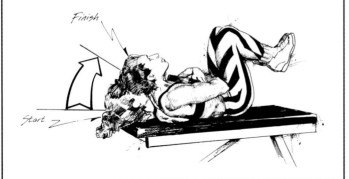

Because of the abdominal musculature's importance to posture and stabilization of the trunk, failure in this case means to the point of losing good form. This boundary can be pushed with the use of a well-trained spotter. A sample beginner program is as follows:

BEGINNER'S PROGRAM

COORDINATION	SETS	REPS	REST	TIMES/WK.
LOWER ABDOMINAL COORDINATION/STRENGTHENING				
1. SUPINE PELVIC TILT	2-6	TO FATIGUE OR LESS THAN 2 MIN./ SET	1:00	7
2. SUPINE PELVIC TILT SINGLE LEG	2-6	TO FATIGUE OR LESS THAN 2 MIN./ SET	1:00	7
3. SUPINE PELVIC TILT UNSUPPORTED	2-6	TO FATIGUE OR LESS THAN 2 MIN/ SET	1:00	7
4. COORDINATION/STRENGTH EXERCISE SUPINE PELVIC TILT - 1/2" KNEEUPS	1-3	5-35	2:00	1-3
OBLIQUE STRENGTHENING				
ALTERNATING CROSS CRUNCH	1	10-30	2:30	3
UPPER ABDOMINAL STRENGTHENING				
STANDARD CRUNCH	1	10-30	1:00	3

Perform exercises at a slow tempo: three seconds concentric, three seconds eccentric. Add resistance when able to perform maximum number of reps indicated.

Former bodybuilding competitor Sharon Bruneau flexes her beautiful abdominals during competition.

INTERMEDIATE PROGRAM

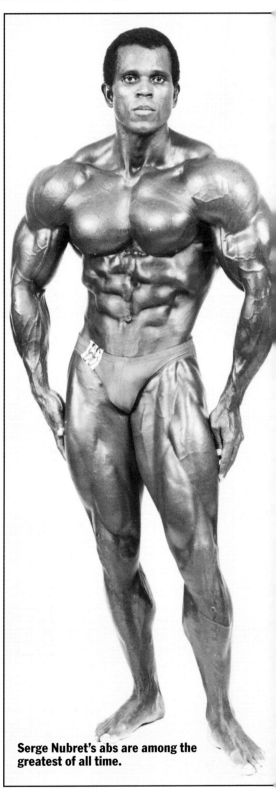

LOWER ABDOMINAL	SETS	REPS	REST	TIMES/WK.
REVERSE CRUNCH – HORIZONTAL PLANE WHEN 3X15 CAN BE PERFORMED PROGRESS TO EXERCISE 3	1-3	10-15	1:30	3
REVERSE CRUNCH – PROGRESSIVE INCLINE	3	8-12	1:30	3
OBLIQUES				
CROSS CRUNCH – PELVIC COUNTERROTATION	3	10-20 ea. side	2:00	3
ALTERNATING CROSS CRUNCH CAN BE DONE ON INCLINE AS WELL	3	10-20 ea.side	2:00	3
UPPER ABDOMINAL				
STANDARD CRUNCH WITH INCLINE	3	8-12	1-1:30	3

Perform exercises at a slow tempo: three seconds concentric, three seconds eccentric. Add resistance when able to perform maximum number of reps indicated.

FIGURE 25 Crunch With Weight on Incline

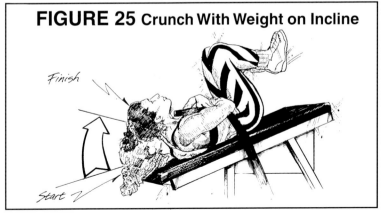

Finish

Start

Serge Nubret's abs are among the greatest of all time.

ADVANCED PROGRAM

LOWER ABDOMEN	SETS	TEMPO	REPS	REST	TIMES/WK.
HANGING REVERSE CRUNCH	3-5	102	6-15	2:00/4:00	2-3
REVERSE CRUNCH – PROGRESSIVE INCLINE	3	313	8-12	1:00	2-3
OBLIQUES					
*SEATED TORSO ROTATIONS WITH CABLE	3-5	313	12-20	L-R 2:00	2-3
*LOWER-BODY ROTATIONS WITH CABLE	3-5	102	12-20	L-R 2:00	2-3
UPPER ABDOMEN					
STANDARD CRUNCH ON INCLINE WEIGHTED	3-5	323	6-12	1:00	2-3
CABLE-RESISTED CRUNCH	3-5	323	6-12	1:00	2-3
AND / OR					
CRUNCH MACHINES	3-5	203	6-12		2-3

NOTE: *Any additional exercises from the menu can be added to the routine for those desiring more work than the advanced program offers. Remember in such cases, though, that the back and abdominal muscles must not be allowed to become unbalanced. If this begins to happen, a bent-forward posture with a forward head and rounded shoulders often develops. This posture is common among wrestlers and boxers.*

Tempo formula: The numbers are in the order of the exercise movements. The second number is a hold number. For instance, in the reverse crunch the first number, 3, means the crunch is performed for 3 seconds. The next number is 1, which represents a 1-second hold. The third number, 3, indicates that the eccentric phase of the reverse crunch is performed for 3 seconds.

WHEN TO INCREASE WEIGHT: *Add resistance when able to perform maximum number of reps indicated.*

*To tone and slim the obliques, use the indicated rep/ set/ rest prescription. To build mass, switch to 8-12 reps, 3-5 sets, slow tempo, and rest less than 60 seconds between sets.

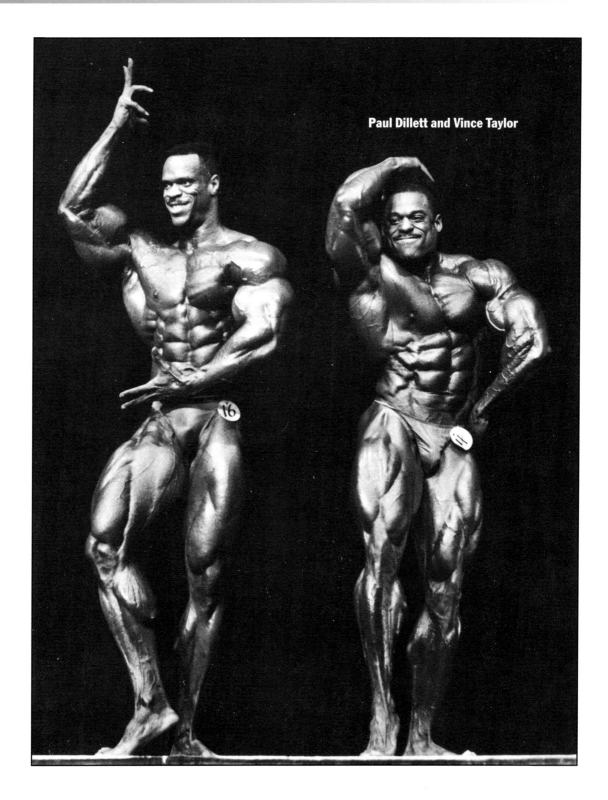

Paul Dillett and Vince Taylor

EXERCISE MENU

COORDINATION	LEVEL	FREQUENCY
SUPINE PELVIC TILT (Exercise 1)	1	DAILY
SUPINE PELVIC TILT- SINGLE LEG (Exercise 2)	2	DAILY
SUPINE PELVIC TILT - UNSUPPORTED (Exercise 3)	3	DAILY
SUPINE PELVIC TILT - 1/2" KNEEUPS (Exercise 4)	3	DAILY unless muscle soreness develops
LOWER ABDOMEN		
SUPINE PELVIC TILT - UNSUPPORTED *Knees at 90° or more	1	daily
REVERSE CRUNCH - HORIZONTAL PLANE	2	2-3
REVERSE CRUNCH -PROGRESSIVE INCLINE	3	2-3
HANGING REVERSE CRUNCH	4	2-3
OBLIQUES		
ALTERNATING CROSS CRUNCH	1	2-3
CROSS CRUNCH WITH PELVIC COUNTERROTATION	2	2-3
SEATED TORSO ROTATION WITH CABLE	4	2-3
LOWER-BODY ROTATION WITH CABLE	4	2-3
UPPER ABDOMEN		
STANDARD CRUNCH	1	2-3
CRUNCH WITH INCLINE	2	2-3
CRUNCH WITH WEIGHT	3	2-3
CRUNCH WITH WEIGHT AND INCLINE	3	2-3
CABLE-RESISTED CRUNCH	3	2-3
CRUNCH MACHINES	3	2-3

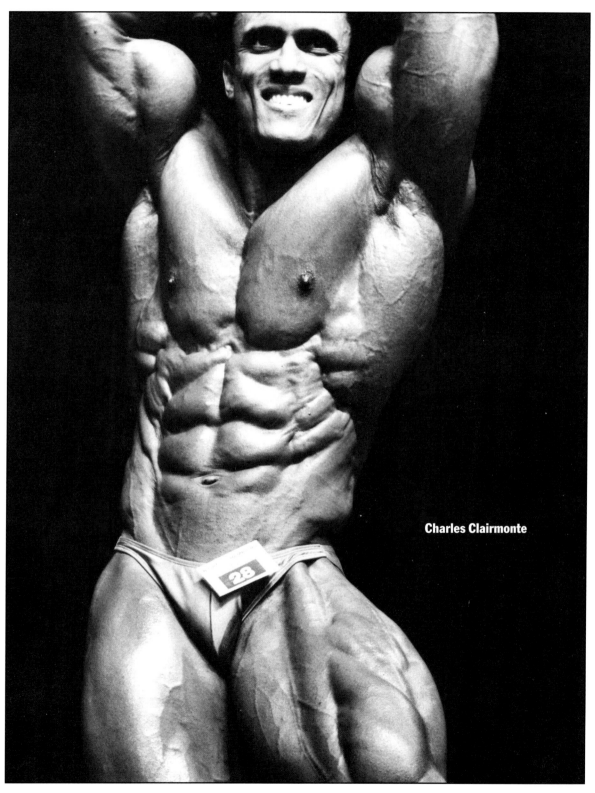

Charles Clairmonte

Although many fitness enthusiasts work their abdominals diligently, few can be seen stretching these important muscles. The abdominal muscles, like all striated skeletal musculature, are susceptible to shortening with repeated hard workouts. There are not only postural implications to such neglect, but the normal excursion of the ribs during breathing is altered. This change encourages use of neck muscles to aid in the breathing cycle and is commonly associated with muscle-tension

FIGURE 26
Crunch on Incline With Weight Belt

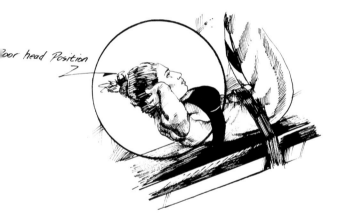

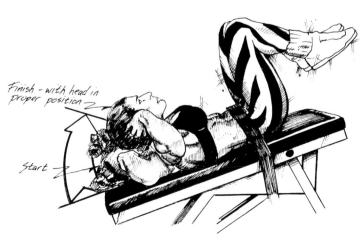

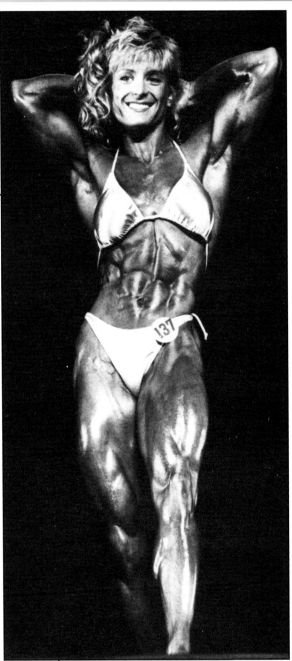

Sue Price is proud of her magnificent midsection.

headache. To avoid such consequences, I highly recommend stretching as shown in Fig. 23 after every abdominal strengthening session.

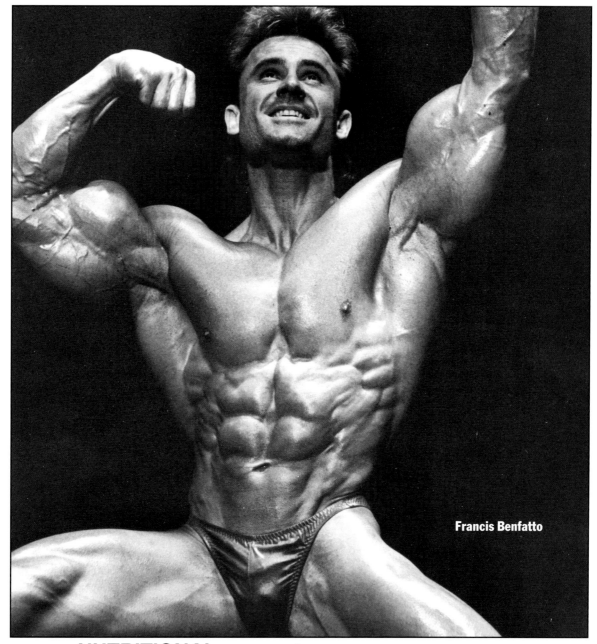

Francis Benfatto

NUTRITIONAL CONSIDERATIONS FOR AWESOME ABDOMINALS

Although I have heavily emphasized function in this manual, I'm sure a majority of readers are very interested in aesthetics as well. The only way a well-coordinated, well-developed abdominal region can be appreciated by yourself and others is to be free of any excess fat that may be covering it.

The fact is, most who are involved in recreational conditioning/weight training have both poor diets and a limited understanding of what is required to properly nourish an exercising body. Because there are many good books available on sports nutrition today, our emphasis will be on a few of the key nutritional components involved with being healthy while developing your washboard abdomen.

The number one diet change must be a reduction of your dietary fat intake (often a large reduction). This is not only a healthful maneuver, but also the catalyst to success if you have been training hard for some time and feel that there may be a well-defined abdomen hidden under the fat. A reduction in dietary fat is often the difference between looking soft and hard, or in the degree of definition you possess.

In this day and age fat is hidden everywhere in our diets. If you were to make a gallant effort to remove all fat from your diet, you would be very unlikely to ever reduce your bodyfat content to a harmful level.

Fat reduction means calorie reduction since a gram of fat is equal to nine calories and both protein and carbohydrate are worth only four calories per gram. From this fact alone we can see that reducing fat consumption will encourage weight loss as fat loss, not by water loss or muscle-wasting as often results from poorly managed, sporadic diets.

In his excellent book *Fit or Fat Target Diet*, Covert Bailey makes the following suggestions

Aaron Baker, Lee Labrada and the late Andreas Munzer.

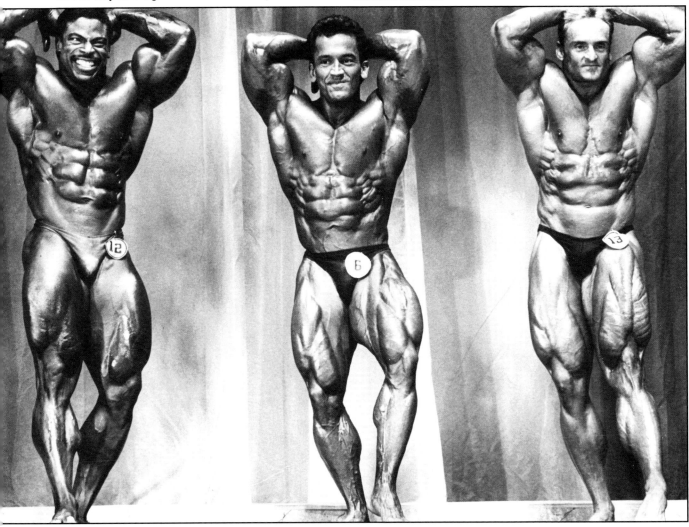

on reducing fat in your diet:

1. Purchase low-fat, low-sugar items if possible (preferably without artificial sweeteners).

2. Reduce or remove butter and margarine whenever possible. If nothing else, see how little you can get by on. A low-calorie butter substitute

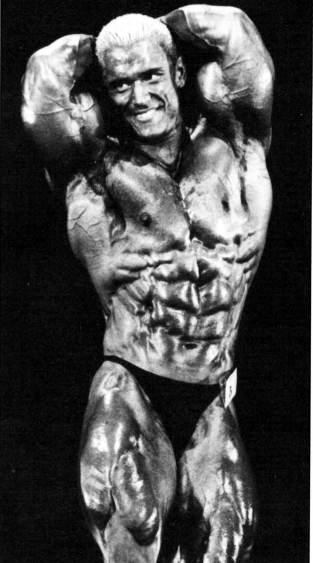

Lee Priest hits a fabulous ab pose.

called Butter Buds can be purchased in most grocery stores.

3. Trim all fats off meat before cooking, not after. Fat soaks into meat during the cooking process, saturating the meat with unwanted calories.

4. Remove the skin from fish and poultry before cooking. The skin contains a lot of fat (calories!).

5. Avoid frying food. If it is a must, use a stick-free frying pan to prevent having to use fat to reduce sticking.

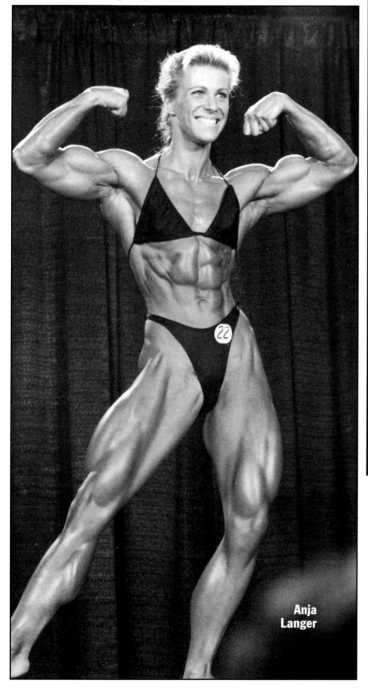

Anja
Langer

6. Bake, steam, broil, or use a wok when cooking. None of these requires grease for the cooking process.

7. Wean yourself from whole milk by mixing it 50/50 with 2 percent, and then use the same technique to reduce to skim milk.

8. Buy only low-fat cottage cheese and hard cheeses.

9. Eat ice milk or low-fat frozen yogurt in place of ice cream. These products often taste good enough that you may not even miss ice cream.

10. When buying meat, ask the butcher which cuts are low in fat content. Some examples are flank steak, round steak and veal.

11. Avoid roasted nuts. Most of the nutrients are destroyed in the roasting process. Raw nuts contain much more nutrition per calorie. Remember that a large percentage of the calories in nuts comes from fat!

12. To avoid topping potatoes with butter, try using soup, or even low-fat salad dressing mixed 50 percent with plain low-fat yogurt.

13. Mix salad dressings with plain yogurt 50/50.

14. Avoid sweetened cereal. You will be amazed at how great natural grains (pearl

Kevin Levrone, Dorian Yates and Shawn Ray in competition.

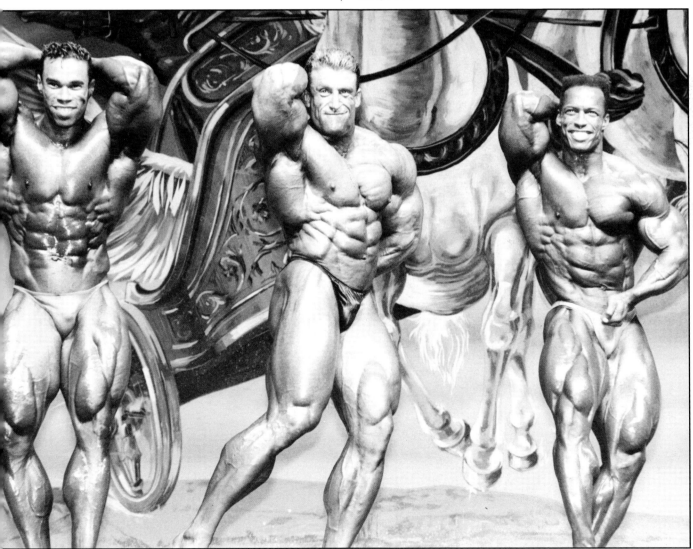

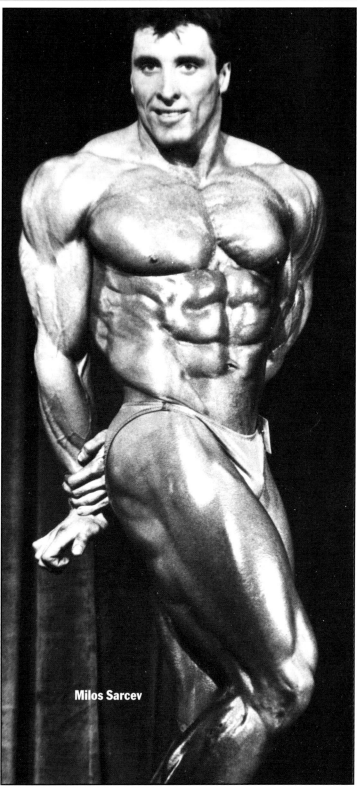

Milos Sarcev

barley, whole red wheat, whole oats, etc.) taste when boiled with a little unsulfured dry fruit mixed in. Once you try these cereals, you will never want the processed garbage again.

15. Purchase water-packed, not oil-packed canned goods whenever possible.

16. Snack on foods like celery sticks, carrot sticks, low-fat yogurt, plain popcorn, fresh fruit, and bagels without fattening toppings, instead of empty calories like chocolate bars, cookies and junk food in general.

17. Eat your fill on nutritious calories before you eat any dessert foods (empty calories.)

18. Eat until full, not until it hurts!

19. Avoid fattening processed spreads such as mayonnaise and artificial cheese spreads.

20. When purchasing breads always get the 100 percent whole-grain products (wheat, rye, 8 grain etc.). Because whole grains are high in fiber, the calorie content is often lower because a portion of the grain is indigestible, and some of the calories just pass right through.

21. Replace bacon and pork sausage with low-fat chicken or turkey sausages or turkey bacon.

22. Try low-sugar, lower-butter syrups in place of regular high-fat, high-calorie types.

23. Instead of eating dessert every night, try using a dessert as a reward for reaching a short-term goal.

24. Avoid deep-fried fast foods. They are high in fat content.

25. Request that items like grilled potatoes be cooked dry (without oil), and that toast be delivered with butter on the side. Often these items are drenched with unwanted fat calories.

PROTEIN CONSIDERATIONS

The building blocks of our bodies are protein. For any individual maintaining an athletic lifestyle, protein requirements will be increased in proportion to his/her level of physical activity. Recently many sources of nutritional literature have emphasized that

North Americans are eating as much as five times their daily protein requirement. This has led to a reduction in the amount of protein eaten by both athletes and nonathletes.

James Webber M.D. (of San Diego, CA) frequently emphasizes the need for adequate protein consumption, which he feels is one gram per kilogram of bodyweight per day, with athletes often requiring more than that. He goes on to point out that not only physical stress, but also mental stress (e.g. job, financial, relationships) causes increased need for protein.

A lack of protein may carry many consequences according to Dr. Webber. He states that today we have more aesthetically conscious males and females than ever. Unfortunately they are eating rabbit food and taking part in as much as two hours

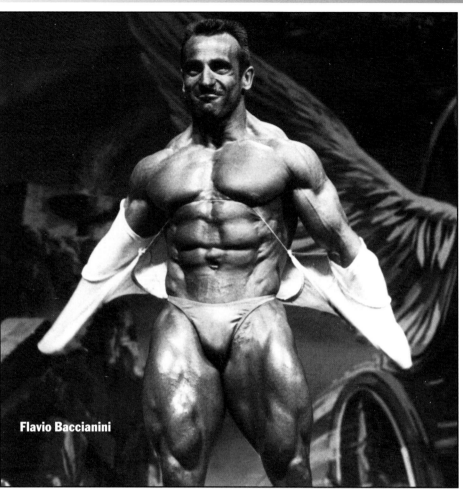

Flavio Baccianini

of exercise or more a day. Because of stress, poor dietary habits (e.g. lack of fiber), and even frequent use of some medications, many of our intestinal tracts are unable to properly digest and absorb protein. Famous Canadian strength coach Charles Poliquin says that each gram of meat (i.e. beef, poultry, etc.) contains only .23 grams of protein. In this case one gram of meat per kilogram of bodyweight may not be enough to supply the body's demands. The individual who is eating the normal amount for his bodyweight will be faced with marginal deficiency symptoms.

In the athletically active individual common symptoms of protein deficiency include slow recovery from exercise, lack of motivation, and heightened sense of pain and discomfort. Both the athlete and nonathlete can suffer from

symptoms such as fatigue, reduced ability to concentrate, moodiness, decreased memory, reduced quality of sleep, and even a diminished sex drive.

With these facts in mind it becomes clear that a prerequisite to building a washboard abdomen, or any muscle for that matter, is sufficient protein intake. There is a drive to advertise the use of isolated amino acids in many of the bodybuilding circles today. This is not a necessary endeavor for the active fitness enthusiast. According to Tim Katke of Metagenics in San Clemente, CA, the body is equipped to break protein down into single amino acids as it needs them, in the exact amounts it needs. In an attempt to create a product that provided the highest-quality protein that was easily assimilated, Mr. Katke states that

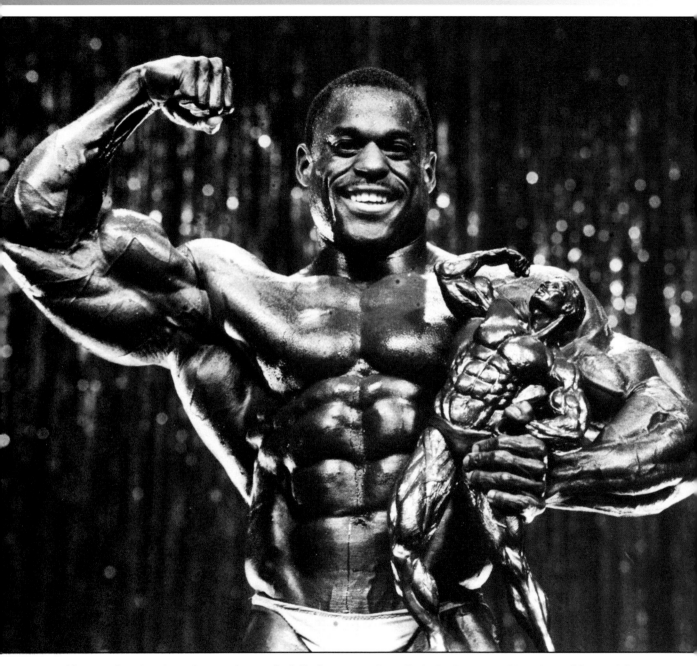

Vince Taylor's abs are nothing short of fantastic!

Metagenics developed a product called Endura Optimizer, which uses Lactalbumin, a milk-and-egg protein that is already broken down so that the body can easily digest it, thus improving absorption. Lactalbumin is predigested and seldom causes an allergic reaction.

The dietary sources of protein should not be overlooked either. There is so much to be said for getting protein from both animal and nonanimal sources. Some good sources of animal protein are egg whites, lean beef, skin-free chicken or turkey and white fish. By adding items such as low-fat cottage and hard cheeses, and low-fat yogurt, you can effectively enhance your daily protein intake. There are many sources of protein in vegetables, grains and legumes. These sources are often incomplete (not containing all the essential amino acids), but provide a complete source when eaten together. A good example of this combination is that of rice and beans, either of which is incomplete alone but which provide a complete source of protein together.

A sample day's eating may look like this:

BREAKFAST
Oatmeal, pearl barley, or winter (red) wheat boiled with unsulfured, unsweetened dry fruit bits, topped with skim milk and/or low-fat yogurt.

LUNCH
Tuna, turkey, skinned chicken, or lean beef sandwich with whole-grain bread and lettuce, tomato and onions (as you desire).
Carrot sticks and/or celery sticks, and two rolled-oat cookies with raisins.

DINNER
Black beans and long-grain brown rice, a tossed salad with low-calorie dressing, a serving of halibut or equivalent white fish, and orange juice. Dessert could be nicely taken care of with low-fat frozen yogurt.

For a detailed look at the anatomy and exercises you can order my video *Scientific Abdominal Training*, available now in advanced and basic versions. Also available is my all-exercise ab video. For video orders, correspondence courses, consulting, video production or seminars call Paul Chek's Center for Health and Performance at 1-800-552-8789 or 619-551-8787.

Paul Chek can be reached at Paul Chek's Center for Health and Performance, 565 Pearl St. #108, La Jolla, CA 92037.

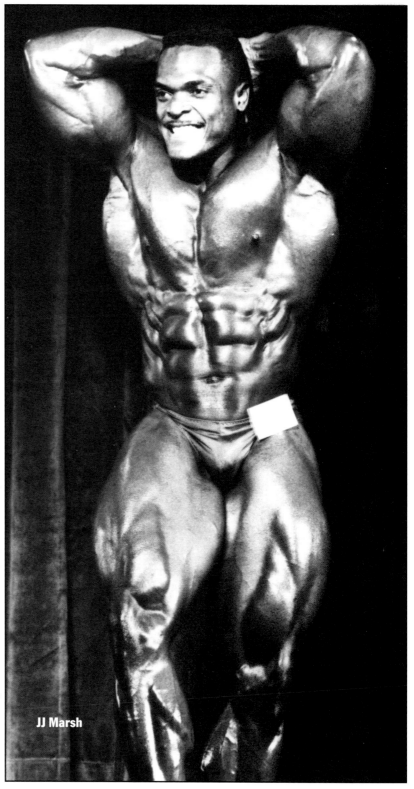
JJ Marsh

GLOSSARY

Accessory respiratory muscles: muscles other than the diaphragm and abdominal musculature which may be used for forced breathing. The muscles include the upper trapezius, sternocleidomastoid, scalenus and levator scapula muscles.

Aesthetics: beauty in appearance.

Anterior: front

Cervical: indicating the portion of the spine which makes up the neck.

Dynamic stabilization: the ability to stabilize one segment of the body such as the pelvis while moving another segment such as a leg.

Endura Optimizer: the name of a nutritional supplement.

Exacerbate: to make worse.

Extensors: muscles that straighten joints.

Flexors: muscles that bend joints.

Forward head and/or forward head posture: the forward migration of the head relative to the shoulder, hip and ankle joints in an upright standing position or seated position.

Hydraulic support mechanism: used interchangeably with intra-abdominal pressure.

Hyperactive: indicating spasm or excessive use of a muscle group or muscles.

Hyperflexing: exaggerated bending of a joint or joints.

Hypertrophy: an increase in size of muscle.

Inspiration: the act of inhaling.

Internal and external obliques: the muscles along the outer edges of the rib cage. These muscles flex and rotate the trunk. The external oblique rotates the trunk to the opposite side while the internal oblique rotates the trunk to the same side.

Intra-abdominal pressure: pressure within the thoracic cavity or rib cage that aids in decompression of the lumbar spine during lifting maneuvers.

Lactalbumin: a predigested protein product.

Legumes: vegetables of the bean family.

Lesser trochanter: a protuberance on the inner aspect of the hip at which the psoas (major hip flexor) attaches.

Lumbar curvature: the arc of the lower back.

Lumbar spine: the lower five segments of the spine.

Microtrauma: very small areas of trauma to soft tissues in the body, used here to refer to trauma to muscles from exercise.

Pelvic counterrotation: rotation of the pelvis in the opposite direction to the torso.

Pelvic tilt: the tilting motion of the pelvis. Picturing the pelvis as a bowl, anterior pelvic tilt would have the fluid pouring out of the front of the bowl, while the posterior pelvic tilt would have fluid pouring out of the back of the bowl.

Physiological: indicating normal function of the body.

Postural degeneration: a worsening of one's posture.

Rotators: muscles that rotate joints.

Spondylolisthesis: the forward slippage of one vertebra on top of another, most commonly found in the lower lumbar segments of the spine.

Sternum: chest bone.

Synergistically: working together.

Thoracolumbar fascia: a broad sheet of connective tissue in the lower back region that has muscle fibers from the latissimus dorsi, internal oblique and transverse abdominus muscles attaching to it. This connective tissue acts as a support system for the lower spinal region.

Tonus: the resting tension in a muscle.

Vector: an intersection of lines denoting a distance or a coordinate axis.

INDEX

– CONTRIBUTING PHOTOGRAPHERS –

Josef Adlt
Garry Bartlett
Robert Kennedy
Chris Lund
Jason Mathas